Reverse Type 2 Diabetes

How to Control and Prevent Diabetes Naturally

By

Kim Hilton

Reverse Type 2 Diabetes

First edition. May, 2018.

Copyright © 2018 Kim Hilton

Written by Kim Hilton

Books by The Same Author

- <u>How to Get Rid Of Stretch Marks Naturally</u>

- <u>How to Break Sugar Cravings with Nutritional Supplements:</u> Healthy and Natural Alternatives

- <u>The Anti-Anxiety Cookbook:</u> Nutritional Plan to Cure Depression and Anxiety (Stress Relief and Mental Health Cookpot)

- <u>Eating Disorder Recovery Workbook:</u> How to Recover from Eating Disorder On Your Own (Anorexia, Bulimia Nervosa, And Binge Eating)

- <u>100 Health Hacks Nobody Ever Told You:</u> Natural Tips and Tricks for Enhanced and Prudent Well-Being

- <u>How to Lower Blood Pressure Naturally & Quickly:</u> Powerful Tricks to Deal with Hypertension Using Supplements and Other Natural Remedies

Table of Contents

Introduction

Diabetes mellitus commonly known as diabetes is a chronic disease that affects millions of people around the world; it is characterized by high levels of sugar in the blood and it comes with three main symptoms which are frequent urination (polyuria), frequent hunger (polyphagia) and increased thirst (polydipsia).

Statistics shows that more than 382 million people have diabetes worldwide; its main cause is insulin problems, for now, there is no cure but the condition can be managed effectively.

We have three common types and they are type I diabetes, type 2 diabetes which will be looking at and gestational diabetes. Pre-diabetes is a condition where someone has high levels of sugar in the blood but not high as that of diabetes.

This raises the risk for any of the three types of diabetes; prevention and early diagnosis is the best way to prevent full blown diabetes.

Type I diabetes is caused by the inability of the body to produce insulin; it is also known as insulin-dependent diabetes, early-onset diabetes or juvenile diabetes. Those with type I diabetes take insulin injections for as long as they live. This type is less common.

Gestational diabetes occurs only in females during pregnancy; it is estimated that 18 out of 100 women experience this during pregnancy, it occurs when there is high levels of sugar in the blood and the body cannot make sufficient insulin to absorb all of it.

Type 2 Diabetes

In type 2 diabetes, insulin is produced but it is not sufficient; it also occurs when the cells of the body cannot respond to insulin (another name for this is insulin resistance diabetes).

90% of diabetic cases worldwide are type 2 diabetes; it is progressive and gets worse over time and the patient is usually required to take insulin tablets. There are natural alternatives to help reverse this condition naturally.

Risk Factors/Causes

Below are some of the causes and risk factors for type 2 diabetes.

- Obesity

- Unhealthy diet

- Sedentary lifestyle

- Regular intake of soda and other sugary drinks

- Genetics and family history

- Age

- Race (People from the middle East, Africans and South Asians have higher risk of type 2 diabetes than any other race)

- Hormonal imbalance

- Heart disease

- Inflammation in the body

- High blood pressure

- Chronic stress

- Exposure to toxins, harmful chemicals and pathogens

- Medication; they are some medications that affect the production of insulin.

Signs and Symptoms of Type 2 Diabetes

It possible to have type 2 diabetes for years and not know it; this is because it shows general symptoms and there are not specific. Below are the main symptoms of insulin resistance diabetes.

- Chronic fatigue

- Blurred vision

- Dizziness

- Frequent and severe thirst

- Frequent urination especially at night

- Slow healing of wounds and cuts

- Unexplained weight loss

- Loss of muscle bulk

- Frequent infections or episodes of thrush

- Irritability

- Itchy skin

- Swollen, red and painful gums

- Frequent gum infections/disease

- Sexual problems in men

- Tingling and feeling of numbness in the feet and hands

Health Complications

Health Complications caused by type 2 diabetes

When diabetes is left untreated; a lot of health problems and complications can arise and they include:

- Cataracts, glaucoma, diabetic retinopathy and other eye complications.

- The inability of the stomach muscles to work properly

- Gangrene, neuropathy, ulcers and other foot complications that may require amputation.

- Skin infections, skin problems and skin disorder

- Heart problems

- High blood pressure

- Mental problems like depression and anxiety

- Ear problems and loss of hearing

- Ketoacidosis

- Gum disease

- Nerve damage that can lead to many problems

- Hyperosmolar hyperglycemic non-ketotic syndrome which is an emergency condition.

- Uncontrolled high blood pressure which leads to kidney disease in most cases

- Peripheral arterial disease

- Erectile dysfunction

- Stroke

- Slow healing wounds

How to Reverse Type 2 Diabetes Naturally

Type 2 diabetes can be prevented and it can also be reversed; this is done by lifestyle changes and healthy diet. The steps listed below will reverse this condition in the natural way and without side effects and it will also help one regain his/her health.

1. Stop eating unhealthy foods

Unhealthy foods are one of the main causes of type 2 diabetes; they cause lots of harm in the body, they trigger inflammation and disrupt immune functions and this can trigger immune response. The first and important step in reversing diabetes in a natural way is to stop the intake of these foods and remove them completely from your diet.

Some of the unhealthy foods to avoid are:

Refined sugar: This is a harmful product that can cause health problems; it increases blood glucose concentration because it can enter the bloodstream rapidly. Avoid taking white refined sugar, soda, fruit juices, sweetened foods and drinks, and even honey and maple syrup.

If you really want to sweeten anything, then use stevia; it does not have much impact on the levels of glucose in the body.

Alcohol: When diagnosed with diabetes; you should try your best to quit alcohol if you drink. It makes the liver toxic and raises the levels of blood sugar.

Grains: These have high amount of carbohydrates, especially the grains that contain gluten like wheat. The body converts large amount of carbohydrates into sugar within a few minutes after eating.

The gluten present in these grains can also cause intestinal problems and inflammation; this can affect the levels of hormones like leptin and cortisol and lead to a high increase in the concentration of blood sugar.

Try and avoid grains for a period of 90 days; this will give your body time to heal, after that you can include sprouted grains slowly and in small amounts into your system.

Dairy: Dairy, dairy products and conventional cow's milk should be avoided and completely eliminated in all its forms; but if you can't and you still need milk, then opt for goat's milk, sheep's milk or milk from A2 cows.

They can help balance blood sugar and they are better than milk gotten from A1 casein cows also known as conventional cows; this milk harms the body, trigger the response of the immune system which is similar to that of gluten.

It is also good you go for organic and raw products gotten from pasture-raised animals.

Hydrogenated oils: This includes cotton seed oil; soybean and canola oil. They give lots of health problems like diabetes because of the manner of process they go through and they also contain chemicals as additives, colorings and bleaching agent agents.

GMO foods: GMO soy, corn and canola gives lots of health problems like diabetes; opt for non-GMO and organic foods.

2. Eat lots of healthy foods

Healthy and organic foods should be your main diet; and this includes:

Fiber rich foods: This helps in reducing the absorption of glucose in the body; it detoxifies the body and regulates the concentration of sugar in the bloodstream.

Try and eat at least 30 grams of fiber daily; good sources of fiber are flaxseeds, chia seeds, vegetables, nuts, berries and avocados.

Magnesium rich foods: Magnesium can regulate blood sugar concentration because it plays a role in the metabolism of glucose; studies have even linked diabetes with a deficiency in magnesium.

Take lots of magnesium rich foods like spinach, black beans, organic and unsweetened yogurt, almonds, chard, and pumpkin seeds.

Foods rich in chromium: Chromium is an essential nutrient that is needed in the metabolism of lipids and carbohydrates; it balances the levels of sugar and improves glucose tolerance. It plays a role in the pathways of insulin by taking glucose to the cells of the body so it can be properly absorbed and utilized for energy.

Natural sources of chromium are broccoli, raw cheese, brewer's yeast, grass-fed beef and green beans.

Low glycemic index foods: These foods cannot cause a rise in blood sugar and they include nuts, seeds, berries, avocados, organic meats, coconut, eggs, raw pastured dairy, vegetables that have no starch and stone fruits.

Avoid high glycemic index foods because they lead to an increase in blood sugar.

Healthy fats: Coconut milk, coconut oil, grass-fed butter, red palm oil, and ghee help to balance the levels of sugar in the body; they also serve as a source of fuel (fats).

Clean protein: Proteins have little effects on the glucose levels and it even slows the absorption of sugar; good sources of proteins are grass-fed beef, eggs, organic chicken, bone broth, lentils and fish caught in the wild.

3. Take vital supplements

Chromium picolinate

Take 200 micrograms of this supplement thrice daily with meals; this will help to improve the sensitivity of insulin and also reduce the levels of lipids like triglycerides and cholesterol.

Fish oil: This improves diabetes markers by raising the levels of good cholesterol while reducing the levels of bad cholesterol and triglycerides. They contain omega-3 fatty acids which are needed for healthy functions of insulin;

this reduces inflammation and boosts insulin tolerance. Take a thousand milligram of the supplement daily.

Cinnamon: Cinnamon is effective in reducing blood sugar and increasing insulin sensitivity; add cinnamon to your meals and drinks and you can also take cinnamon tea daily. You can combine 3 drops of cinnamon essential oil with a teaspoon of coconut oil and use it to massage the abdomen, wrist and other body parts.

Bitter melon extract: It can reduce the levels of sugar and regulates the way the body uses insulin; it also helps in the management of diabetes symptoms like hormonal imbalance, insulin resistance, eye problems, heart problems, damaged blood vessels and kidney problems.

Alpha lipoic acid: This antioxidant converts glucose into fuel for use by the body; it reduces the symptoms of diabetic neuropathy like numbness caused by damaged nerves and weaknesses and it improves insulin sensitivity.

Good sources of this are tomatoes, broccoli and spinach and it can also be gotten via ALA supplements.

4. Exercise

Exercises helps in reducing chronic diseases like diabetes and it can reverse it; it improves blood sugar concentrations and has the ability to prevent and delay type 2 diabetes. It also normalizes blood pressure, cholesterol and lipid levels and boosts the quality of life.

It also helps the body burn fats and builds lean muscles; it should be in your daily routine; 30 minutes of moderate exercise a day is enough. Try stretching and walking; at intervals try cardio like weight training or burst training 3 days weekly, this will increase the fat burning rate and increase insulin sensitivity.

Strength training builds and maintains muscles and this helps to keep blood sugar in the right proportions and it also helps the metabolism of glucose.

5. Follow a good diabetic eating plan

Meet an experienced doctor or a well-learned herbalist or dietician to write a diabetic meal plan for you; this will help you balance the levels of sugar and you will even see immediate results.

You can start with this for now, it is a three days plan; you can add more after consulting with a dietician or nutritionist, stick to this meal plan, try not to cheat and eat as much healthy foods as you can.

Day one

Breakfast: coconut smoothie, add chai or flax seeds, organic powder, cinnamon and stevia.

Lunch: large spinach and chicken salad, dress it with olive oil and apple cider vinegar.

Dinner: Grass-fed beef burger with steamed broccoli.

Snacks: ¼ cups of raw almonds.

Day two

Breakfast: vegetable omelet and goat cheese cooked in coconut oil.

Lunch: chicken vegetable soup with bone broth.

Dinner: wild-caught salmon, sauté it in coconut oil and grill it with spinach and onions.

Snacks: A2 raw cheese

Day three

Breakfast: peach prebiotic drink, made with goat milk, frozen peaches, almond butter, cinnamon and protein powder.

Lunch: small salad and turkey burger.

Dinner: stir-fry made with chicken and vegetables

Snacks: raw veggies and guacamole.

6. Avoid stress and sleep more

All kinds of stress like emotional stress, physical and mental stress raise the levels of sugar, cholesterol and hormones in the body; studies even stated that women who sleep less than 5 hours every day have higher risk of developing type 2 diabetes.

Avoid stress, relax more, sleep at least not less than 8 hours at night and also try to get some naps in the afternoons.

7. Intermittent fasting

A short time without foods helps the body to lower the concentration of sugar; it brings the body back into balance and is beneficial to the whole body.

Fasting triggers a lot of biochemical reactions, like improving insulin sensitivity, reduce sugar cravings, aids weight loss, and lowers the levels of lipids and triglycerides. Fasting speeds up the rate at which the body burns fats and it forces the body to use stored and excess sugar for energy.

Research suggest restricting eating to a specific period of time like 8 am to 8 pm helps the body shift from sugar burning to fat burning. It makes the body use fats as their main source of fuel. If you are on medications, it will be safer to consult your doctor before embarking on a fast.

Books by The Same Author

- <u>How to Get Rid Of Stretch Marks Naturally</u>

- <u>How to Break Sugar Cravings with Nutritional Supplements:</u> Healthy and Natural Alternatives

- <u>The Anti-Anxiety Cookbook:</u> Nutritional Plan to Cure Depression and Anxiety (Stress Relief and Mental Health Cookpot)

- <u>Eating Disorder Recovery Workbook:</u> How to Recover from Eating Disorder On Your Own (Anorexia, Bulimia Nervosa, And Binge Eating)

- <u>100 Health Hacks Nobody Ever Told You:</u> Natural Tips and Tricks for Enhanced and Prudent Well-Being

- <u>How to Lower Blood Pressure Naturally & Quickly:</u> Powerful Tricks to Deal with Hypertension Using Supplements and Other Natural Remedies